HAND FOOT AND MOUTH DISEASE (HFMD)

Prevention, Management And Treatment

Sione Michelson

Table of Contents

Introduction

Chances are you have never heard of the hand foot and mouth disease, or you have but know very little about it.

Hand, foot and mouth disease (HFMD) is a disease of predominantly infants and children under 5 years. Young children in daycare centers, schools and kindergartens and those who attend gatherings with other kids are most susceptible to contracting the disease. It is associated with crowding and poor sanitation and family outbreaks are common.

Here's a quick and comprehensive guide to help you understand the cause, prevention, management, treatment, possible complications and all you need to know about the Hand, Foot and Mouth Disease.

This ebook is intended to be a useful resource for healthcare providers, parents, caregivers or anyone seeking to know more about the HFMD. It contains all you need to know about the disease, the prevention and proven steps and strategies to help treat the disease. For ease of use, throughout this eBook, HFMD, which is the acronym for the disease, will be used interchangeably with Hand, Foot and Mouth Disease.

Chapter 1

What Is Hand Foot And Mouth Disease (HFMD)?

Hand, foot, and mouth disease is a common and highly contagious viral illness that usually affects infants and children younger than 5 years. The illness is not limited to only people of this age as it can occur in older children and adults. It is usually a mild illness which when allowed to run its course, disappears in a few days.

If your child has blisters in and around his/her mouth and a rash on the palms of the hands, soles of the feet and sometimes his/her buttocks and legs, it is likely that he/she has contracted the Hand Foot and Mouth Disease. This disease occurs all year round but most commonly in spring and fall.

You may be familiar with the hoof and mouth disease, that affects livestock and other animals. HFMD is not to be confused with it, as Foot (hoof) and Mouth Disease is an unrelated disease that does not affect humans. HFMD cases were first described in New Zealand in the year 1957. Family outbreaks are common.

What causes HFMD?

The illness is caused by viruses from the Picornaviridae family called the Coxsackie virus. The name "Coxsackie" was derived from the town where this agent was first isolated: Coxsackie, New York.

Coxsackie A16 virus which is a serotype of the virus, is the commonest cause of this illness while Enterovirus 71 is the second commonest cause. Other serotypes of the Coxsackievirus are rare causes.

In HFMD, the source of the infection is "an infected child or adult" meaning people contract this virus from other people. The virus is present in the stool, nasal discharge, blisters/rashes, sputum and saliva of an infected person. The ways of transmission are via the fecal-oral route (through ingestion of the stool or products contaminated with the stool of an infected person) or oral-oral route (through contact with nasal or oral secretions of an infected person).

Fecal material can be ingested by contamination of drinking water supplies, improper handling of diapers and by eating contaminated food. All these occur due to poor hand-washing, poor hygiene and poor sanitation. When an infected person uses the toilet and fails to wash his/her hands properly, he/she may contaminate foods, surfaces or other people's hands and bodies with the virus.

The incubation period, that is the time between exposure to the virus and occurrence of first symptoms, is 3-6 days, on the average.

The following will increase your child's chances of getting infected.

- Playing with neighborhood children
- Visiting hospitals or clinics during epidemics
- Exposure to crowded places.
- Having a weak immune system.

This invariably means that any infant or child can be at risk of contracting this disease. How then can you protect your child from it? Keep reading, as this book will teach you easy ways to prevent the occurrence of this highly contagious disease in your home.

The HFMD is usually a mild illness but in some children, it can run a severe course. Some factors increase the likelihood that a child will have a more severe form of this illness. Some of these factors include (but are not limited to)

- Prior exposure to Epstein-Barr virus. Ebstein-Barr virus is the causative agent of the illness commonly known as the "kissing disease" or "mono".

- Enterovirus 71 infection. Enterovirus 71 has been associated with more severe diseases, greater risks of complications and with epidemics.

- Longer duration of fever.

- Hyperglycemia (elevated blood glucose level) and

- Living in rural areas

Chapter 2

Frequently Asked Questions About HFMD

How common is the HFMD?

The virus is found worldwide and predominantly during the spring, summer and fall months. In the United States, epidemics of Hand-foot-and-mouth disease (HFMD) tend to occur every 3 years. Young children in daycare centers, schools and kindergartens and those who play in public parks and attend gatherings with other kids are highly susceptible to contracting the virus. Also a person, of any age with a weak immune system, is highly susceptible to infection with the virus.

How is the virus transmitted from one person to another?

The virus that cause hand, foot, and mouth disease can be easily transmitted through an infected person's

- Saliva, sputum, or nasal mucus,
- Fluid from the rashes and
- Feces (stool).

It is possible to get the infection or spread it when

- You come in close contact with an infected person- by touching his/her rashes and then touching parts of your body or another person's body, without washing your hands.

- An infected person coughs or sneezes near you or in your face as you may inhale or swallow infected air droplets or the droplets may fall on surfaces and contaminate them.

- You come in contact with an infected person's stool.

- You touch contaminated objects and surfaces like tables and chairs or door knobs. Anyone who touches these surfaces can spread the virus by touching something else.

- You share cups, cutlery, handkerchiefs or face towels.

Other ways of spread include swallowing recreational water contaminated with feces of an infected person (especially if the water has not been properly treated with chlorine), kissing the blistering areas of the face and the mouth and by transmission from an infected mother to her fetus during pregnancy.

Familial exposure predisposes groups of people to infection with the virus. Once the virus is introduced into a household, all susceptible persons usually become infected, although not all will develop symptoms.

A person with hand, foot, and mouth disease is most contagious during the first week of illness. This may continue for days or weeks after all the symptoms have disappeared.

Even if an infected person does not have or show any symptoms, he/she is still able to spread the virus.

HFMD is not?

- caused by being exposed to animals (Hand, foot and mouth disease is not transmitted to or from pets or other animals.)

What happens in your body when you become infected?

As HFMD is an infectious disease, its infectious process, like that of most other infectious diseases can be divided into stages.

Stages of an infectious disease process.

- The first stage is referred to as the "Incubation period". It is the period between when a patient gets exposed to the virus and when the first symptoms of the disease appear. During this period, the virus reproduces or multiplies in the body of the patient and no symptom is present. Sadly, during this period, the virus can be spread, although there are no symptoms. It ranges between 5-6 days.

- The next period is called the "Prodromal period". In this period, nonspecific symptoms appear, that is, symptoms that are not specific for HFMD. The child (or adult) is most infective at this time. It is characterized by fever, weakness, irritability, loss of appetite.

- After this comes the "Illness/Acute period". When symptoms specific for the disease appear. It is characterized by the appearance of vesicles or sores in the mouth, and rashes which occur typically on the palms of the hands and soles of the feet, but can also on other parts of the body.

- The "Declining stage". Here, no new rashes occur and the old ones start to heal. The rashes of HFMD heal without crusting, that is, they do not form a hard outer layer.

- Finally, the "Convalescence period". The patient begins to regain strength. Recovery usually occurs within a week.

HFMD in Pregnancy?

Hand, foot and mouth disease rarely occurs in adults, so the risk of infection during pregnancy is very low. If a pregnant woman contracts the virus in her third trimester, the infection can be transferred to the fetus. Most babies born with hand, foot and mouth disease have only mild symptoms that disappear after a few days.

If a pregnant woman contracts the virus during her first trimester, it may or may not lead to spontaneous abortion or intrauterine growth retardation.

Extra care/precaution should be taken by pregnant women to prevent contracting the virus. Simple hand washing techniques or carrying a hand-sanitizer around can help prevent infection. If you are pregnant and you notice any of the above symptoms (symptoms of infection with the virus) contact your health care provider.

Chapter 3

Signs And Symptoms Of HFM Disease (How You Can Spot A Child With This Disease?)

The HFM disease usually starts with a low-grade fever, sore throat, loss of appetite, abdominal pain and general body weakness. One or two days after the onset of these symptoms, sores in the mouth start to appear. They are first seen, often in the back of the mouth, as small red spots which blister and later ulcerate. If the tongue is affected, in addition to the ulcers, it may be swollen and painful. The appearance of this may be accompanied by loss of appetite, restlessness or crying (in babies) hence, it can often be mistaken for 'teething'.

In older children, they may complain of a sore throat and you may notice a reduction in their appetite. Following the onset of the mouth blisters, rashes start to appear on the palms of the hands and soles of the feet. They may also appear on the knees, buttocks and groin area. The hands are involved more often than the feet, and the back of the hands and sides of the fingers are more commonly involved than the palms.

Usually the lesions in the mouth precede the rash on the skin, but both may occur at the same time.

In severe cases, where there is a complete loss of appetite, dehydration may result, as the child is unable to swallow fluids due to the pain associated with swallowing. If you notice a rash that is similar to what was described above, you should contact your healthcare provider, but do not worry as HFMD is a self-limiting disease, and it should disappear in no time (usually between 7-10 days).

Diagnosis of Hand Foot and Mouth Disease.

A diagnosis is usually made clinically (that is by observing the signs and symptoms). Your health care provider can identify sores and rashes of the hand, foot, and mouth disease and differentiate them from other causes of rashes by considering -

- The age of the patient. If the child is under 5, it can be a major pointer to HFMD.

- The clinical picture of the illness (from onset of symptoms till the healthcare provider sees the child)

- The appearance and healing pattern of the lesion (they heal without crusting- this clinically differentiates them from the vesicles of herpes virus and chickenpox)

- Family and social history (by asking about recent contact with or exposure to a child or an adult with a similar condition)

Remember, not all infected persons will develop symptoms. Some cases are asymptomatic.

Chapter 4

Treatment And Management

There are no specific medications that you can take or give your child to cure hand, foot, and mouth disease. It is usually a self-limiting illness that resolves in 7-10 days. To help relieve symptoms of the illness, some over-the-counter medications can be given to the child or taken by the adult.

- Analgesics like acetaminophen or ibuprofen can be given to ease painful mouth sores or the discomfort from the fever. Aspirin should not be given to children as it may lead to the occurrence of a rare but serious illness called Reye syndrome.

- Mouthwashes or sprays that numb pain in the mouth can be used

- For symptomatic pain control for oral ulcers, elixirs such as benadryl, aluminum and magnesium hydroxide can be helpful. Tell your child to swish the solution in his/her mouth and spit it out, several times daily.

- You can apply topical viscous lidocaine with a cotton swab, several times daily to relieve the pain associated with oral ulcers.

- Calamine lotion may help soothe the rash on the hands and feet.

Antibiotics need not be given to the child as this is a viral infection, but they can be used topically when dressing the wound left behind (after the blisters have ruptured) to prevent bacterial contamination.

This is not a necessary step as the ulcers will heal spontaneously whether or not you do this.

A minority of individuals with hand, foot and mouth disease may require hospitalization due to uncommon neurologic complications such as encephalitis (inflammation of the brain) or meningitis (inflammation of the meninges)

Non-neurologic complications such as myocarditis (inflammation of the heart) or pneumonia may also occur and would require hospitalization. Hospitalization would also be recommended for children that fail/refuse to take anything by mouth. An intravenous line can be set in place and fluids will be given to the child through this.

Management of HFMD (Taking care of a child with HFM Disease.)

Hand foot and mouth disease can usually be managed at home. Only complicated cases will require hospitalization (complications of HFMD will be discussed shortly). Properly feeding and monitoring your child throughout the course of the disease can help prevent these complications or help identify them early enough.

Feeding an infected child and caring for sores/lesions in the mouth.

The most important thing to remember when taking care of an infected child is that he/she needs to drink enough fluids. Due to the presence of sores in the mouth and throat and the irritability and general weakness the child feels, he/she will be unwilling to take in food and sometimes even fluids (especially hot fluids). Hence, dehydration is quite common in children with the Hand, Foot and Mouth disease.

- Dehydration can be prevented by encouraging the child to drink as much fluid as possible especially cold milk or water and not acidic juices, as acidic foods and drinks could worsen the sores. Cold soups and other food which require little effort to consume are good choices.

- Cold yogurt can help sooth the sores and will be enjoyed by your child.

- Giving frozen fruit pops may help to relieve mouth soreness.
- Cereal with cold milk can be given to the child.
- Do not give the child sour or spicy food and drinks.

Caring for the body of an infected child and his/her skin lesions or rashes.

- Lukewarm baths or tepid sponging can help reduce the fever.
- Change the infant's diaper as often as possible because a wet diaper could irritate the blisters and might cause more infection and/or pain. Remember to dispose the soiled diapers properly and to wash your hands after doing this.
- Discourage the child from touching or rupturing the blisters.
- For blisters on the hands or feet, keep the areas clean and uncovered. Wash the skin with lukewarm water, and pat dry.Apply a bit of antibiotic ointment to blisters that burst/pop to help prevent secondary infection (with bacteria) and cover it with a small bandage.
- Try to ensure that the child doesn't play in or with dirt while the sores are still present on his/her body.

When to call/see a doctor

- If the child is very irritable or refuses to take in food or drink, it's time to see your healthcare provider. Call your doctor if your child remains irritable, cries endlessly, is sluggish/weak, or seems to be getting worse.
- If signs of moderate to severe dehydration present. See the doctor if he or she looks dehydrated. Signs of dehydration include a decreased urine output, sunken eyes, sunken fontanelles (soft spot on the baby's head) (try not to elicit this too often) or a dry tongue.

Or If the child has any of the under listed symptoms.

- (Neck stiffness, chest pain, shortness of breath, aversion to light or sound, jerking of the limbs, a very high fever or non resolution or worsening of symptoms).

- If the blisters fail to heal or start to discharge pus (this can be a sign of secondary infection with/by bacteria)

Can a child get re-infected after recovery?

Yes he/she can become infected again, but not by the same virus serotype that infected him the last time. Exposure to a particular virus serotype only provides protection against the infecting serotype. As an example, if a child gets infected with Coxsackie virus A16, he has life-long protection or immunity against it but not against other causes of HFMD like Enterovirus 71, for example. Research is still underway to produce an effective vaccine that can be used against Enteroviruses causing HFMD.

Chapter 5

Prevention Of Hand Foot And Mouth Disease

As of today, there is no vaccine that can protect against the virus that causes HFM disease. A vaccine is still in the works against Enterovirus E-71. HFM disease is highly contagious and can spread through contact with feces, saliva, sputum, mucus from the nose or fluid from the blisters. The following steps should be taken to help prevent the spread of HFMD.

- Frequent and proper hand washing with soap and water is the best protection against HFMD and other infectious diseases. Remind everyone in your family to wash their hands often, especially after using the toilet (make sure you use a clean toilet and keep it clean after use) or changing diapers; before cooking/preparing or eating food and after exposure to or contact with an infected person.

- Shared toys in childcare centers and kindergartens should be cleaned often with a disinfectant solution because many viruses can live on objects for days.

- If you notice that your kid has a fever or blisters on the skin and sores in the mouth, keep him/her home from school or daycare.

- Even after they recover, children can pass the virus in their stool for several weeks, hence the infection can still spread to others, it is not important to let them stay home for some weeks after clinical recovery but proper and adequate hygienic methods should be used.

- Clean and sterilize household/shared utensils properly.

- When a child is infected, it is best if he/she is given a separate set of utensils and dishes till he/she must have recovered and after receiving consent from your health care provider. These utensils should be washed with a different sponge and kept separately.

- Talk with your healthcare provider if you are not sure of when you should return to work or when your child should return to school. The same applies to children returning to daycare.

- -Avoiding close contact such as kissing, hugging, or sharing cups with people with hand, foot, and mouth disease.

- Since HFMD is a contagious disease, it should be reported immediately. Contact your child's pediatrician.

- Early notification of the school or child care center is important. Parents of other children will need to check their kids for symptoms. The classrooms and playrooms would have to be disinfected properly and until these are done, other kids should be advised to stay home, as the virus thrives on surfaces for days.

- Disinfection of contaminated surfaces in the house, such as table surfaces, chairs, walls and floors. Contaminated surfaces should be disinfected using diluted household bleach (you can make this at home by mixing 1 tablespoon of bleach with 4 cups of water). .

- Change and wash the sheets and clothing every day to prevent the virus from spreading.

- To reduce the spread of viruses, do not rupture blisters. Discourage your child from touching or rupturing the blisters or rashes.

- While your child is sick make sure to wipe his saliva if he is drooling a lot as the virus spreads through secretions from the mouth and throat. The towels should be disposed properly and should not be shared. Wash your hands after tending to an infected child.

- People who are sneezing or coughing should cover their mouths. Teach your kid to cough or sneeze in their inner elbow or sleeve.

- Fecal waste and soiled diapers should be handled carefully and disposed properly. Surfaces were the diapers were changed should be kept clean and disinfected after each use.

- Don't allow your child play with his siblings or other kids until his rashes have cleared-up and even a few days after. Ask your doctor about when the "isolation/quarantine" should end.

- Don't allow your child to share fomites with anyone. Fomites are materials and agents which are likely to carry infection and they include towels, toothbrushes, and other personal hygiene products.

Chapter 6

Possible Complications Of The Hand Foot And Mouth Disease.

Health complications from hand, foot, and mouth disease are not common but require immediate medical treatment if present. HFMD caused by Enterovirus E-71 tend to be more severe and can be associated with cardiac and neurologic complications than HFMD caused by Coxsackie A16 and other viruses. The possible complications include:

- Moderate to Severe Dehydration (described earlier)

- Pulmonary edema (accumulation of fluid in the lungs) or pulmonary hemorrhage (bleeding into the lungs) may occur very rarely. They are highly fatal and life-threatening conditions and hence would require urgent medical attention.

- Viral/aseptic meningitis can occur with hand, foot, and mouth disease, but it is rare. Its symptoms include fever, headache, neck stiffness or back pain and would require that the infected person be hospitalized for a few days. The condition is mild and usually has a good prognosis.

- Viral encephalitis (inflammation of the brain) or polio-like paralysis can occur, but it is very rare.

- Pneumonia is also a possible but rare complication. It is associated with fever, shortness of breath (dyspnea), cough and chest pain. It is a possible cause of death in children with HFM Disease.

- Secondary infection of blisters. The blisters can get infected with bacteria particularly when they are touched or scratched often or when they come in contact with dirt. Signs of secondary infection include increased pain or appearance of pain, redness, swelling, slow healing or failure too heal and discharge of pus.

- Fingernail and toenail loss have been reported and are not uncommon. They tend to occur mostly in children within 4-8 weeks after recovering from hand, foot, and mouth disease. The cause and link between HFMD and nail loss is still unclear. If you notice nail loss following HFMD, you need not worry about it as the nail loss is temporary and the nail will grow back without medical treatment.